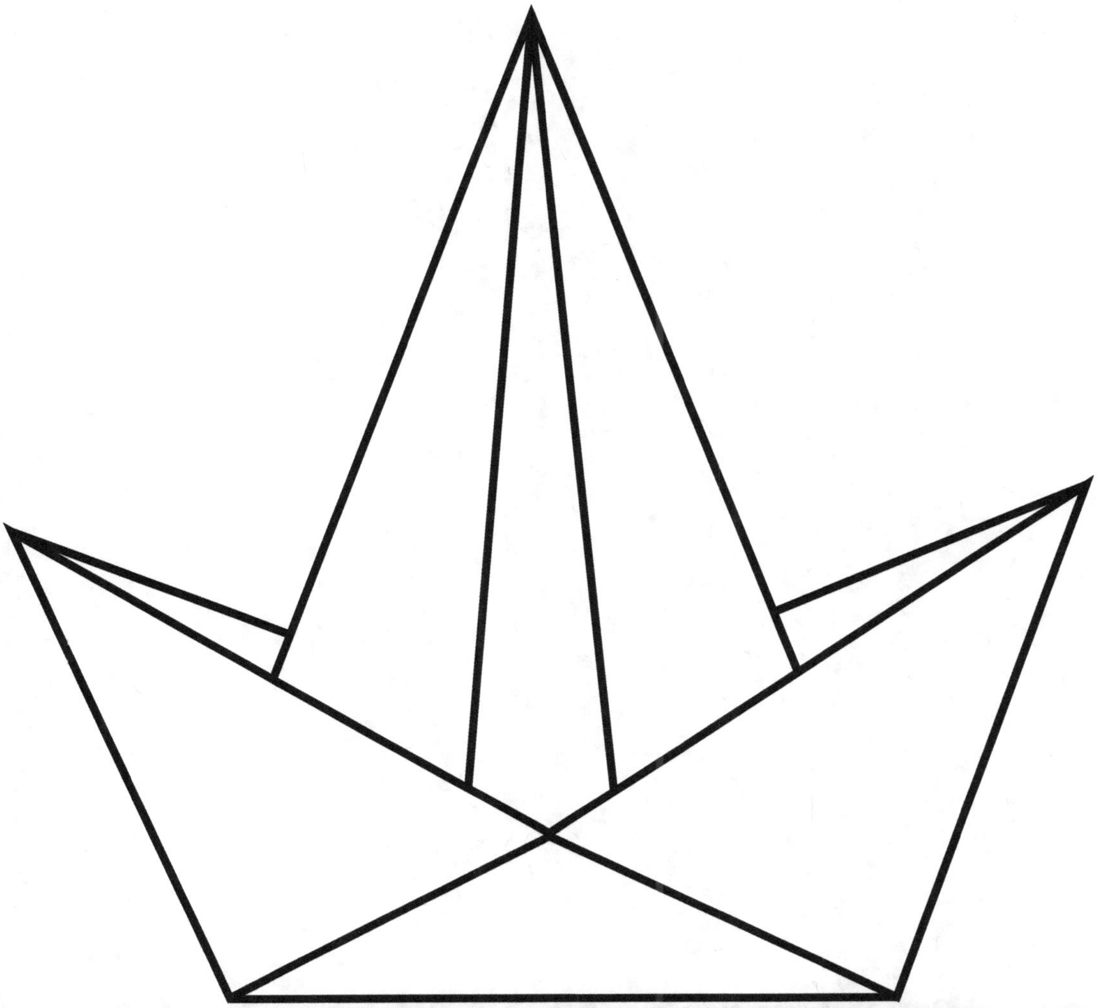

I grew up doing a ton of coloring
books.

They still bring me so much happiness,
which is why I thought it would be fun
to make one of my own.

I hope this brings you some joy.

-Maura

@mauralapesada

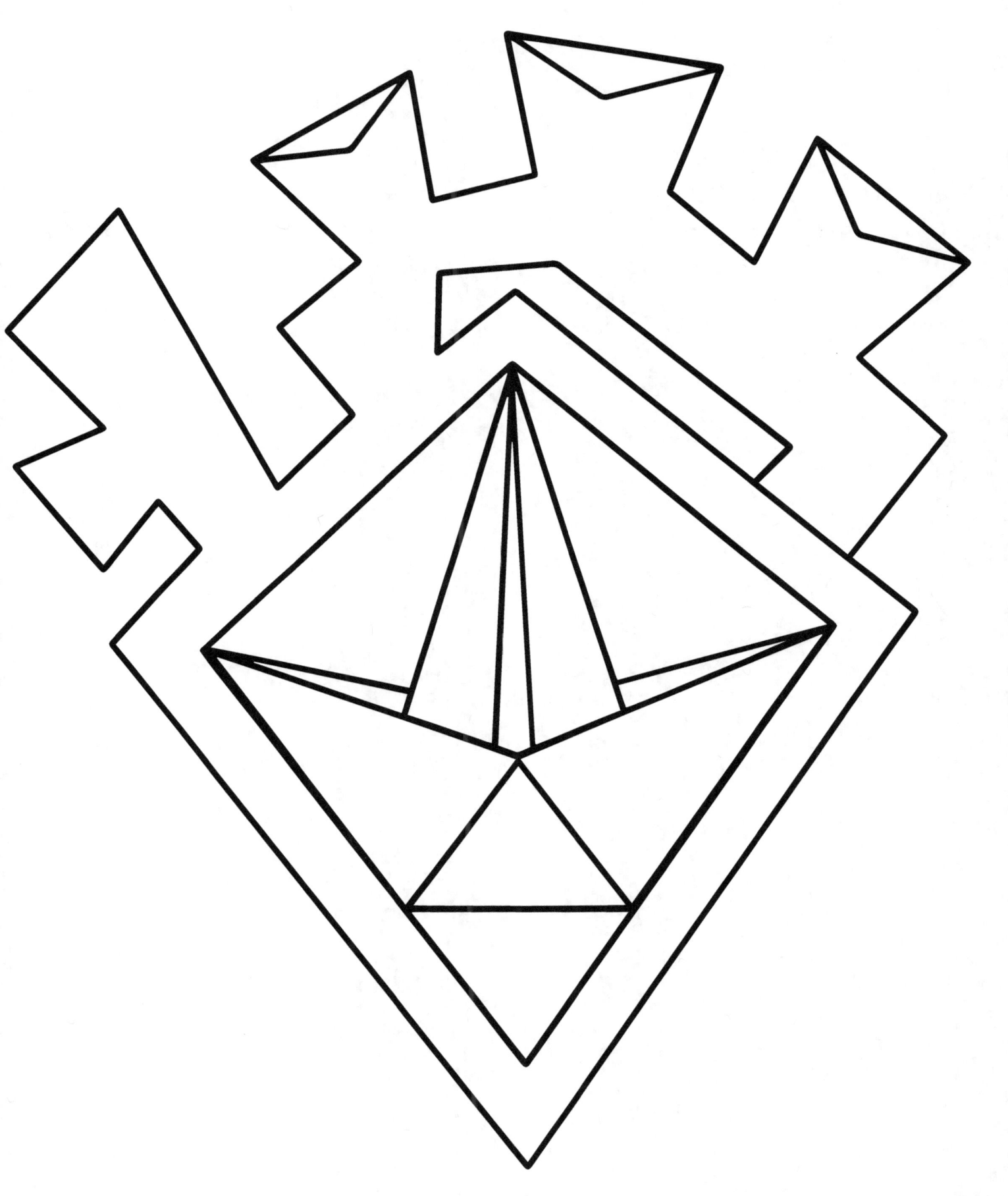

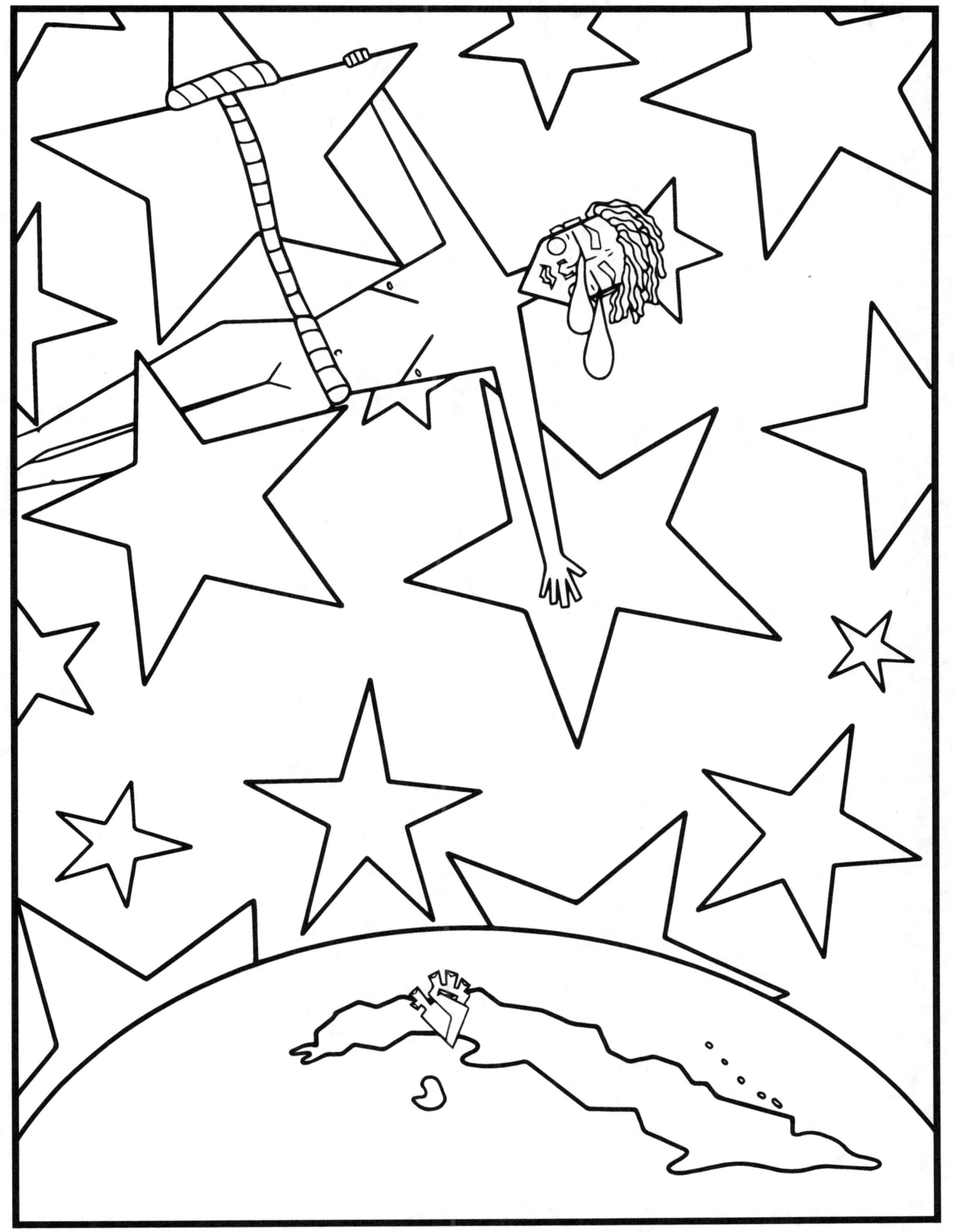

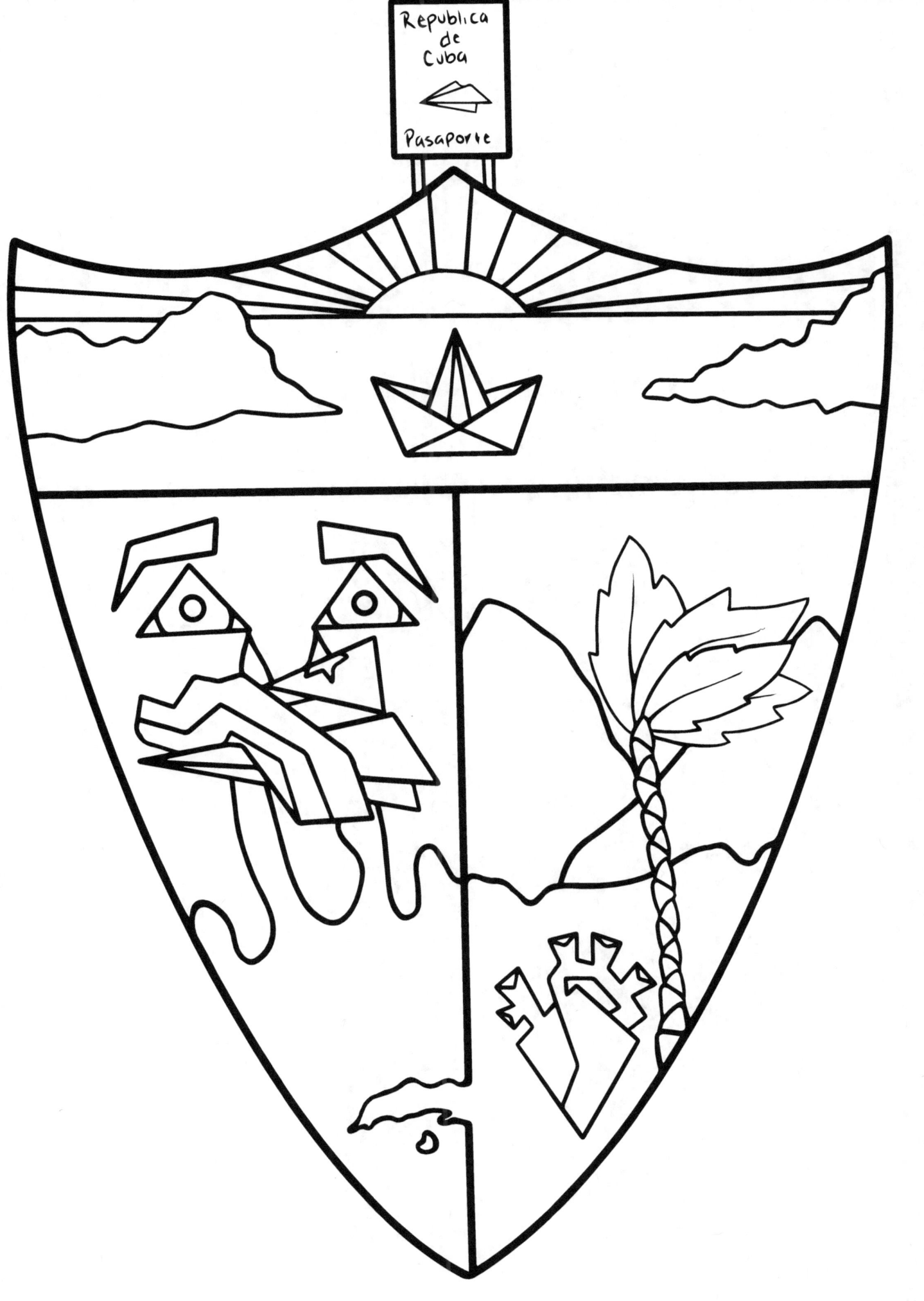

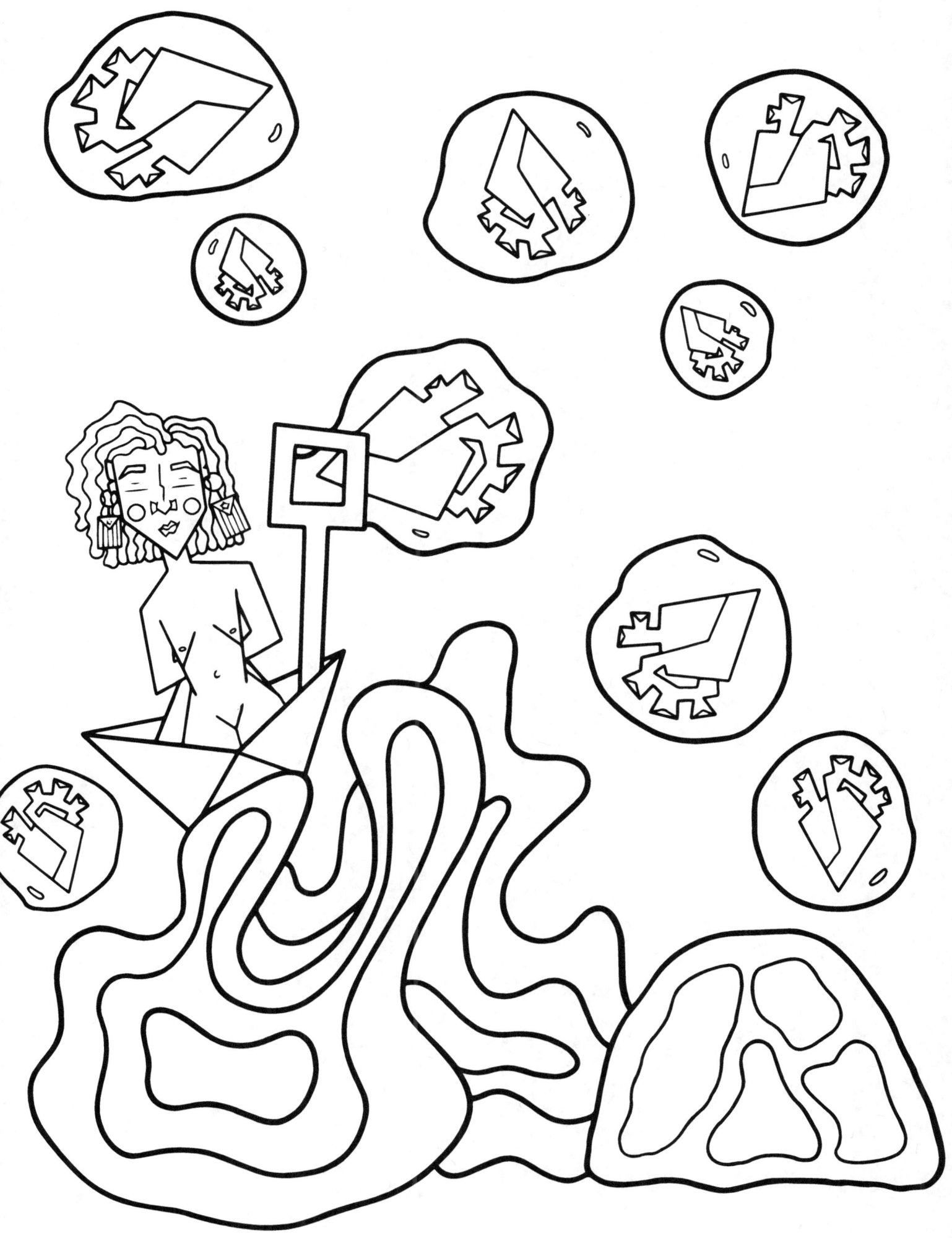

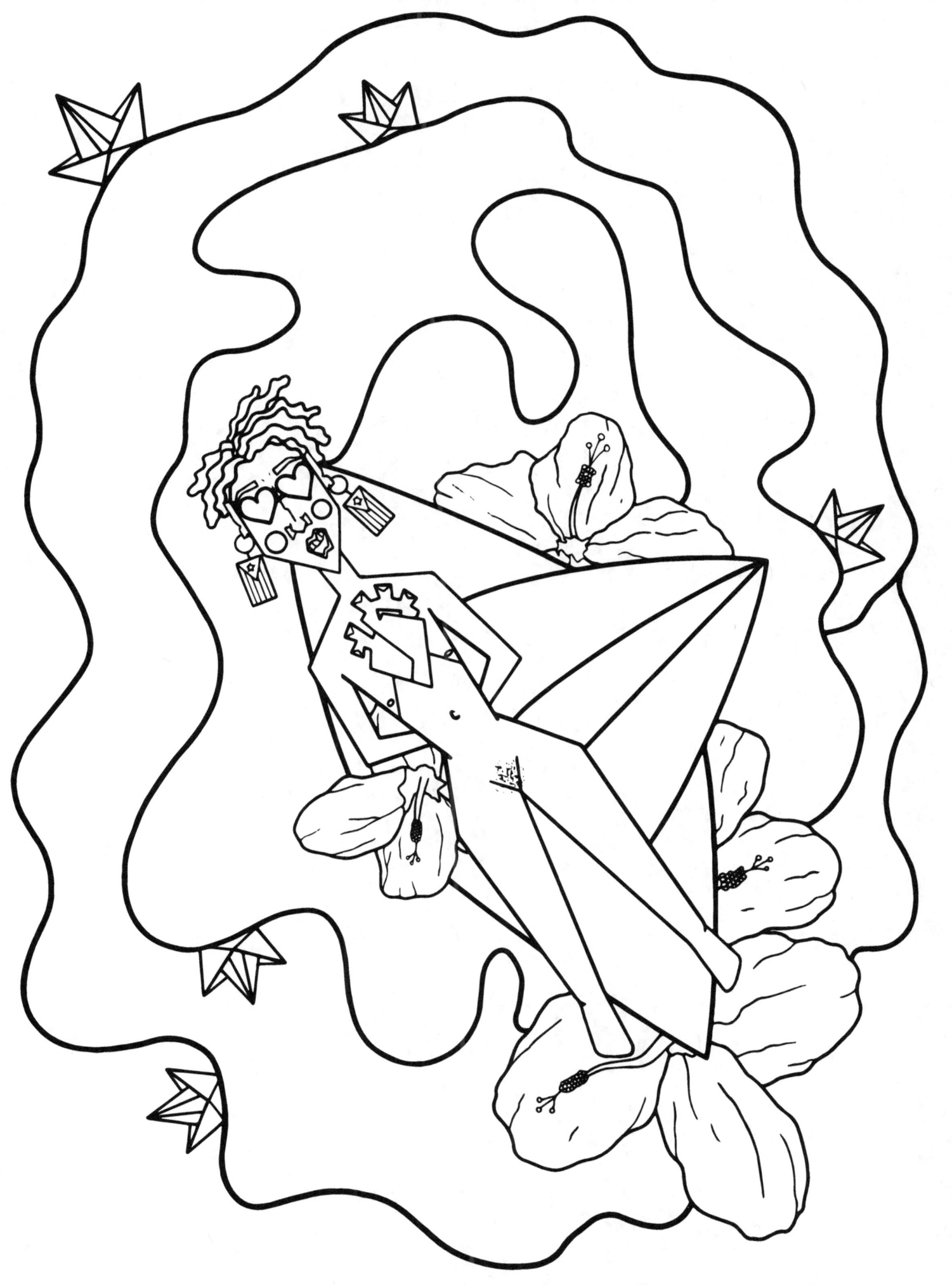

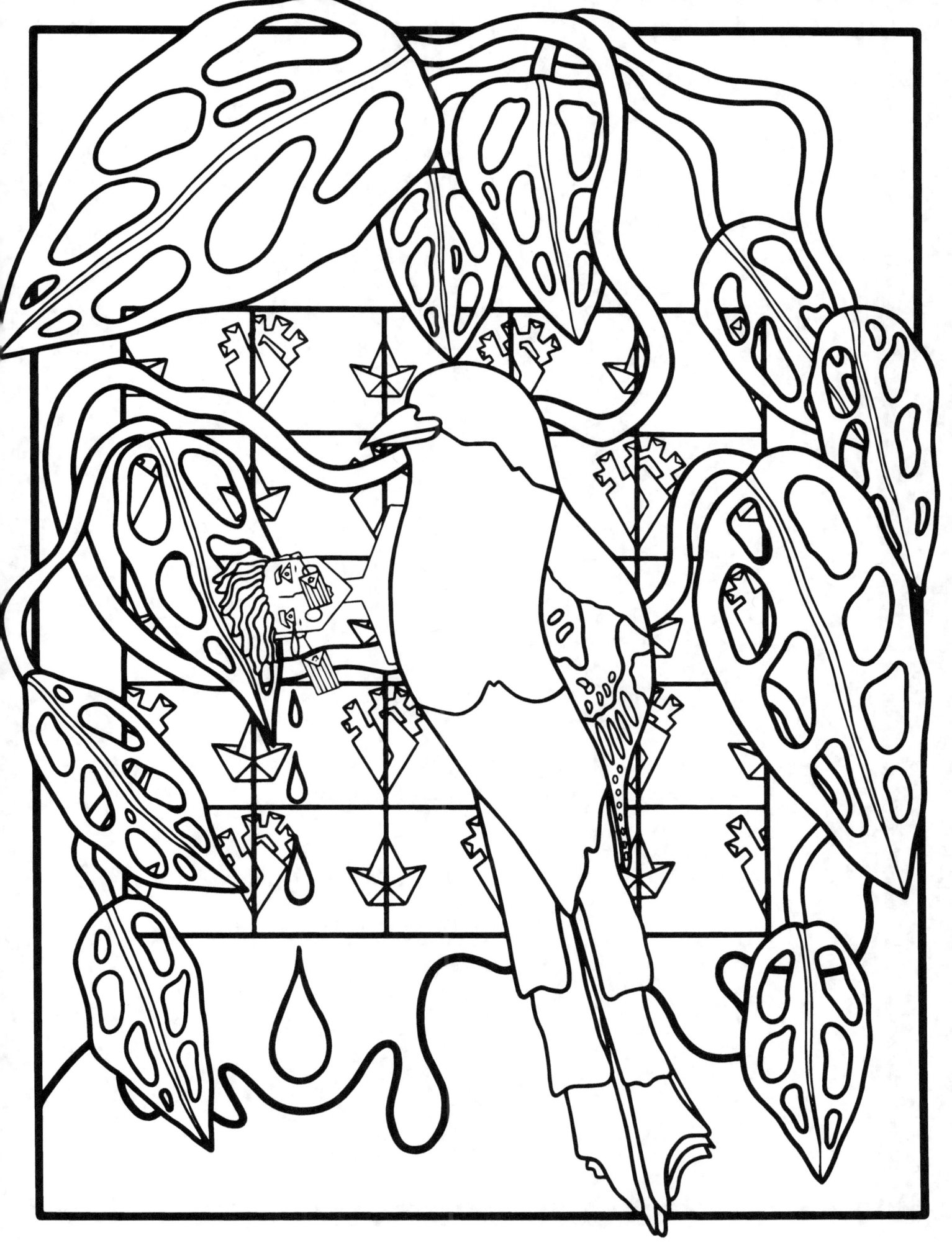

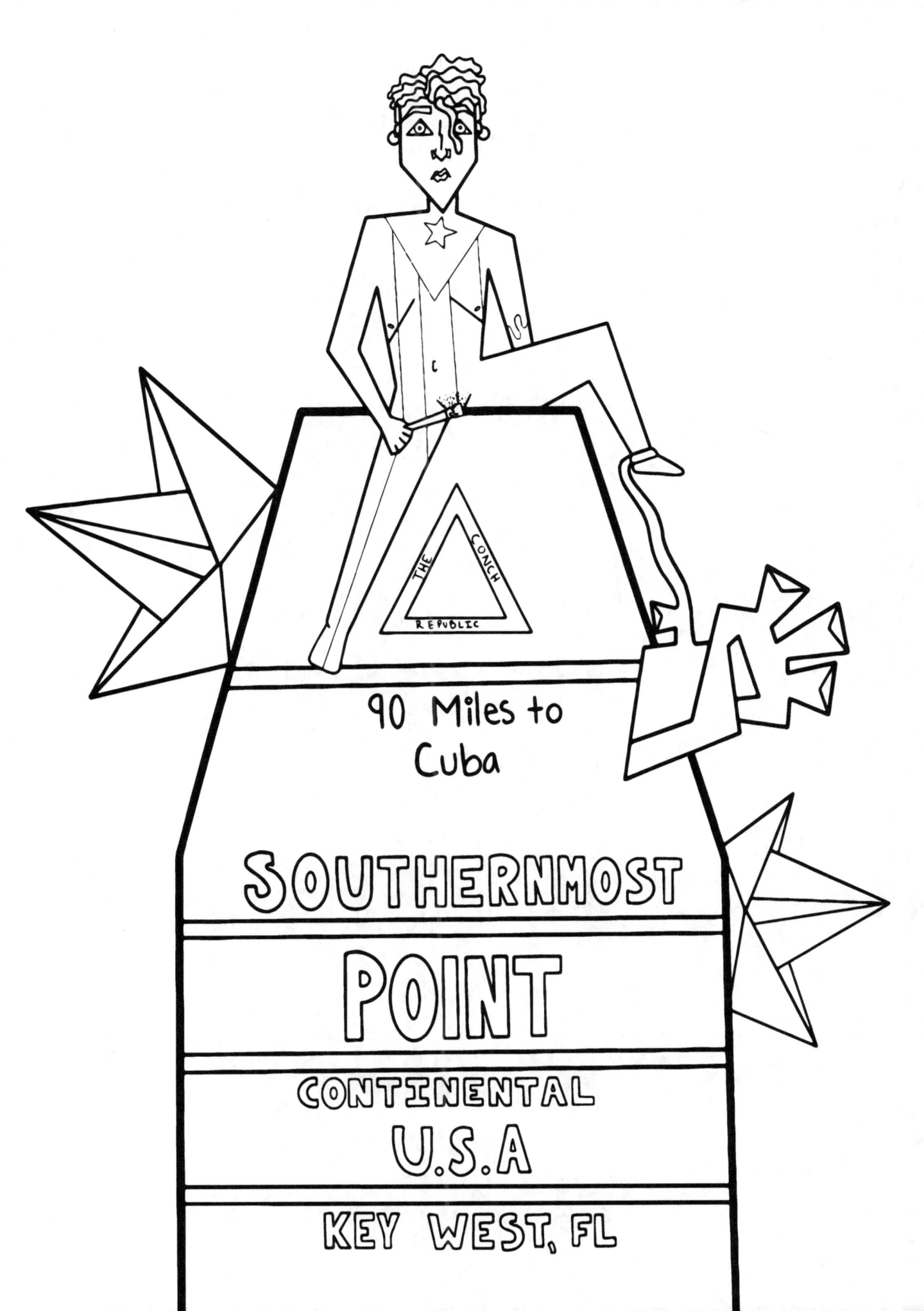

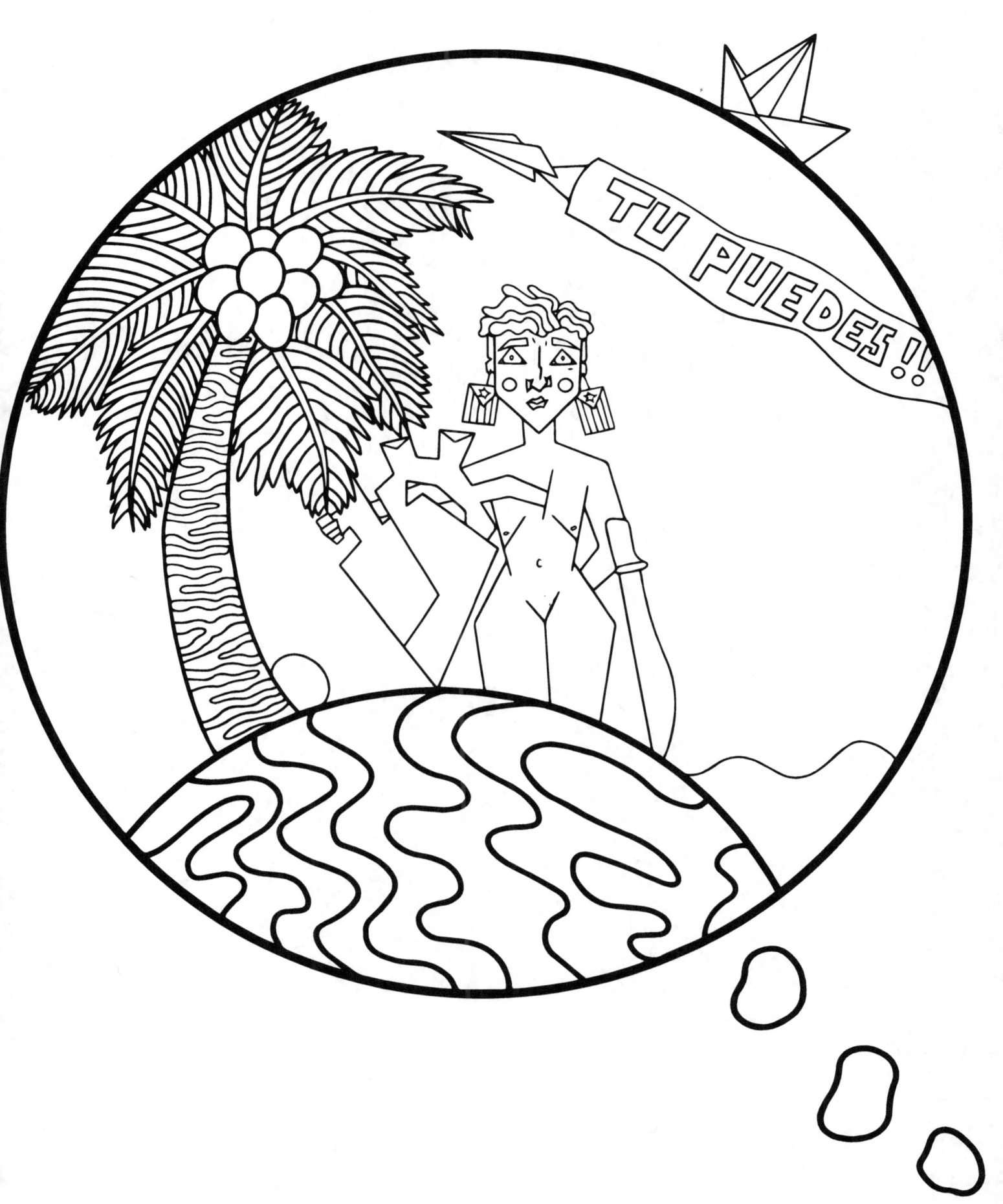

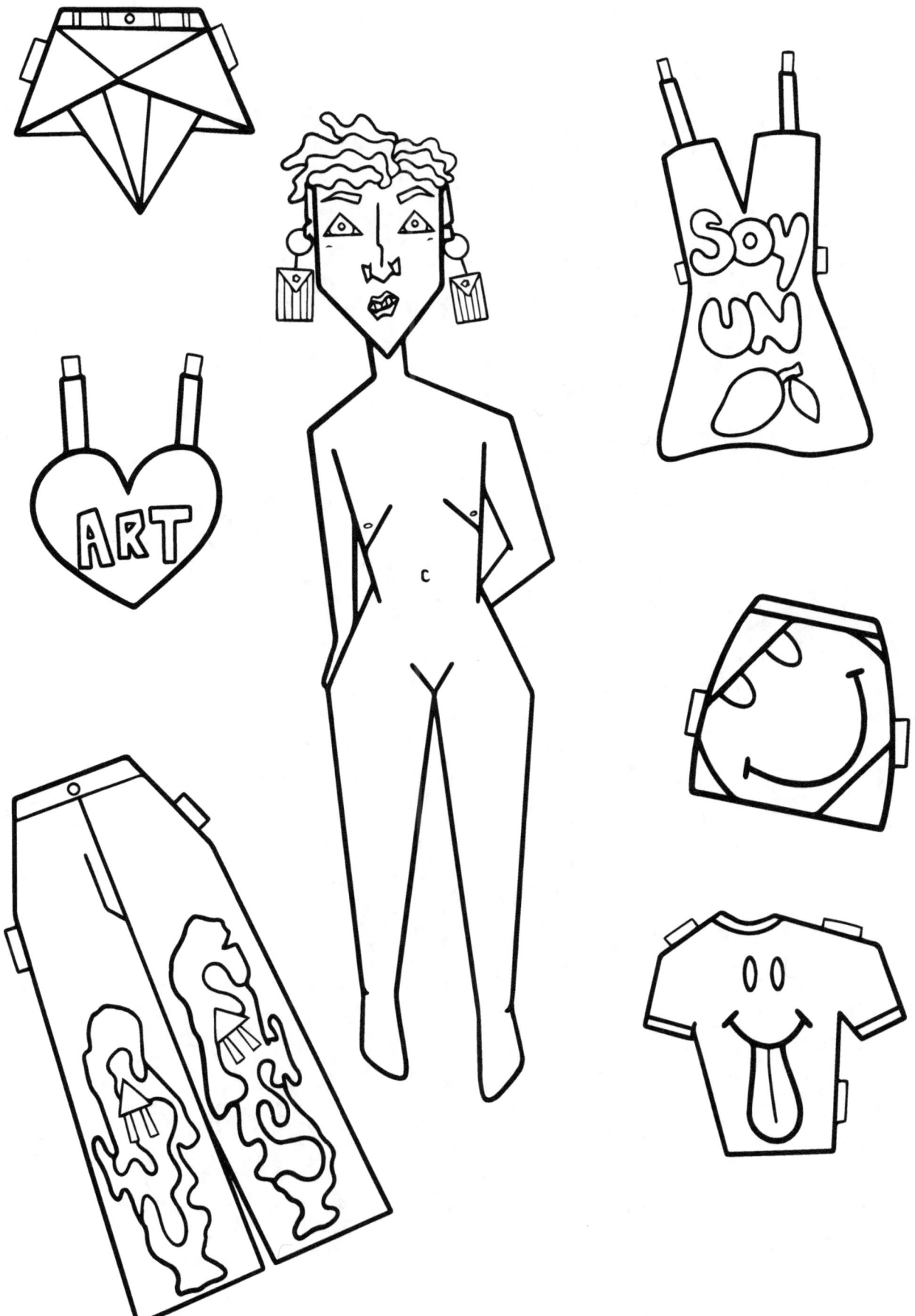

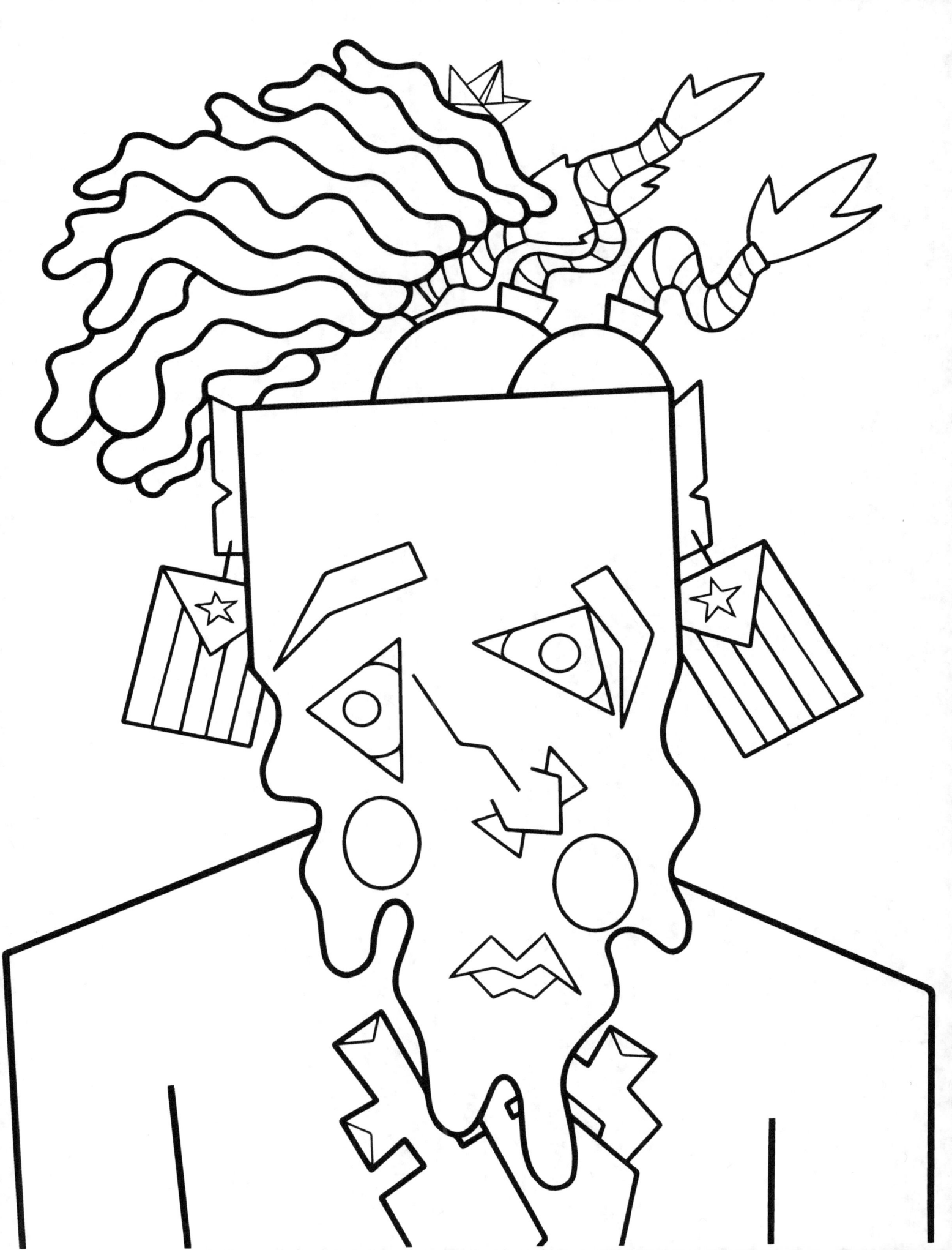

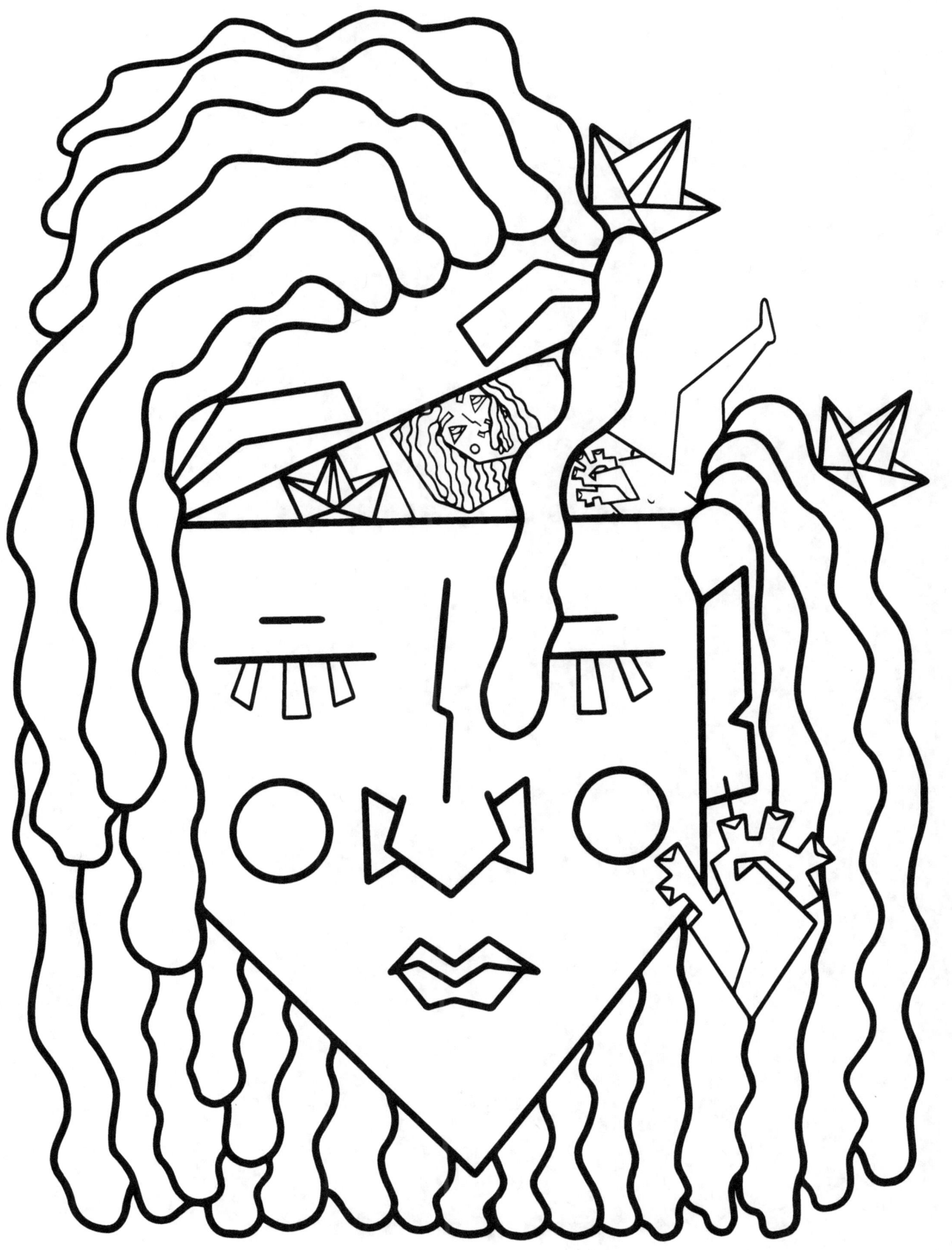

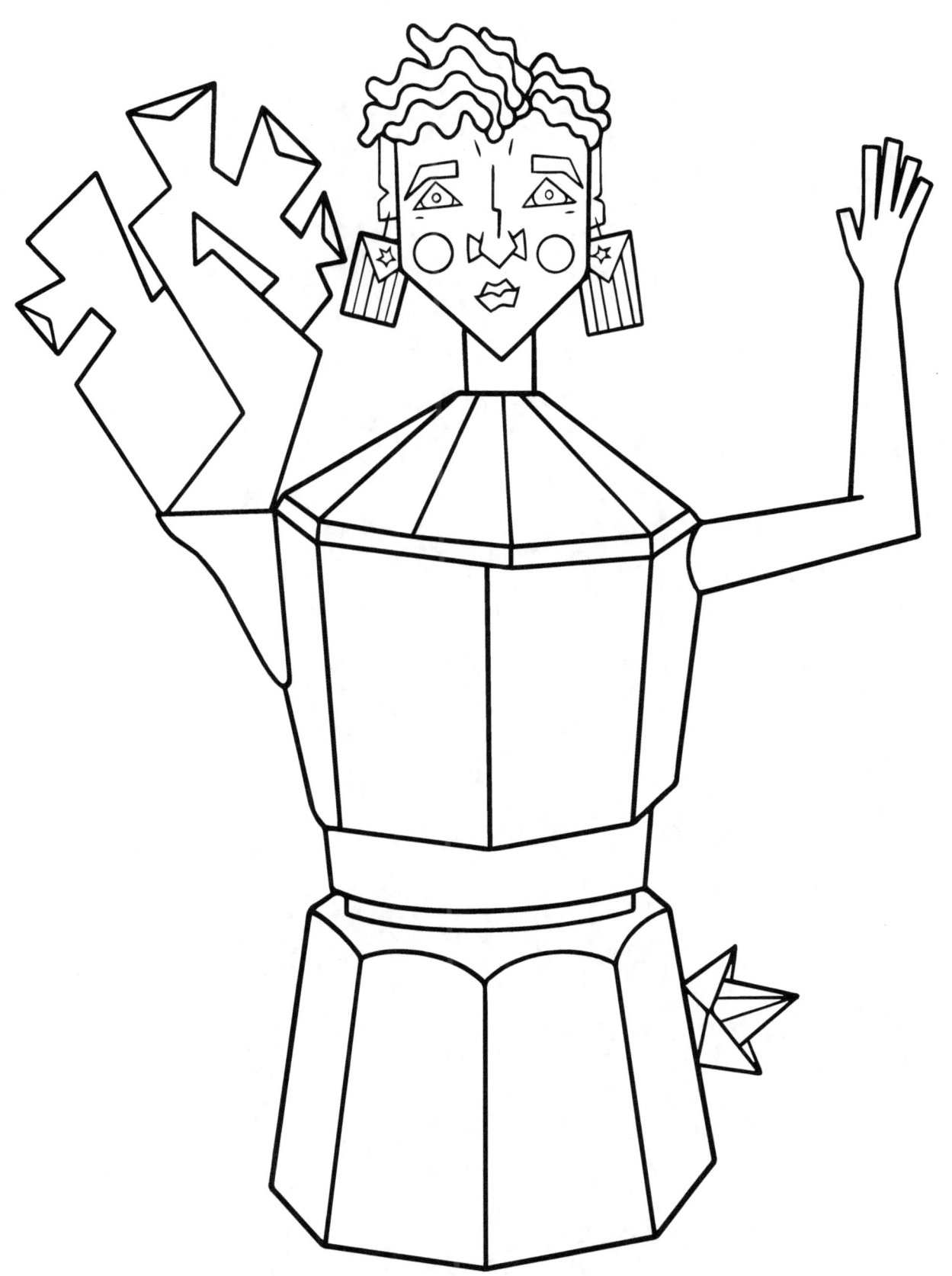

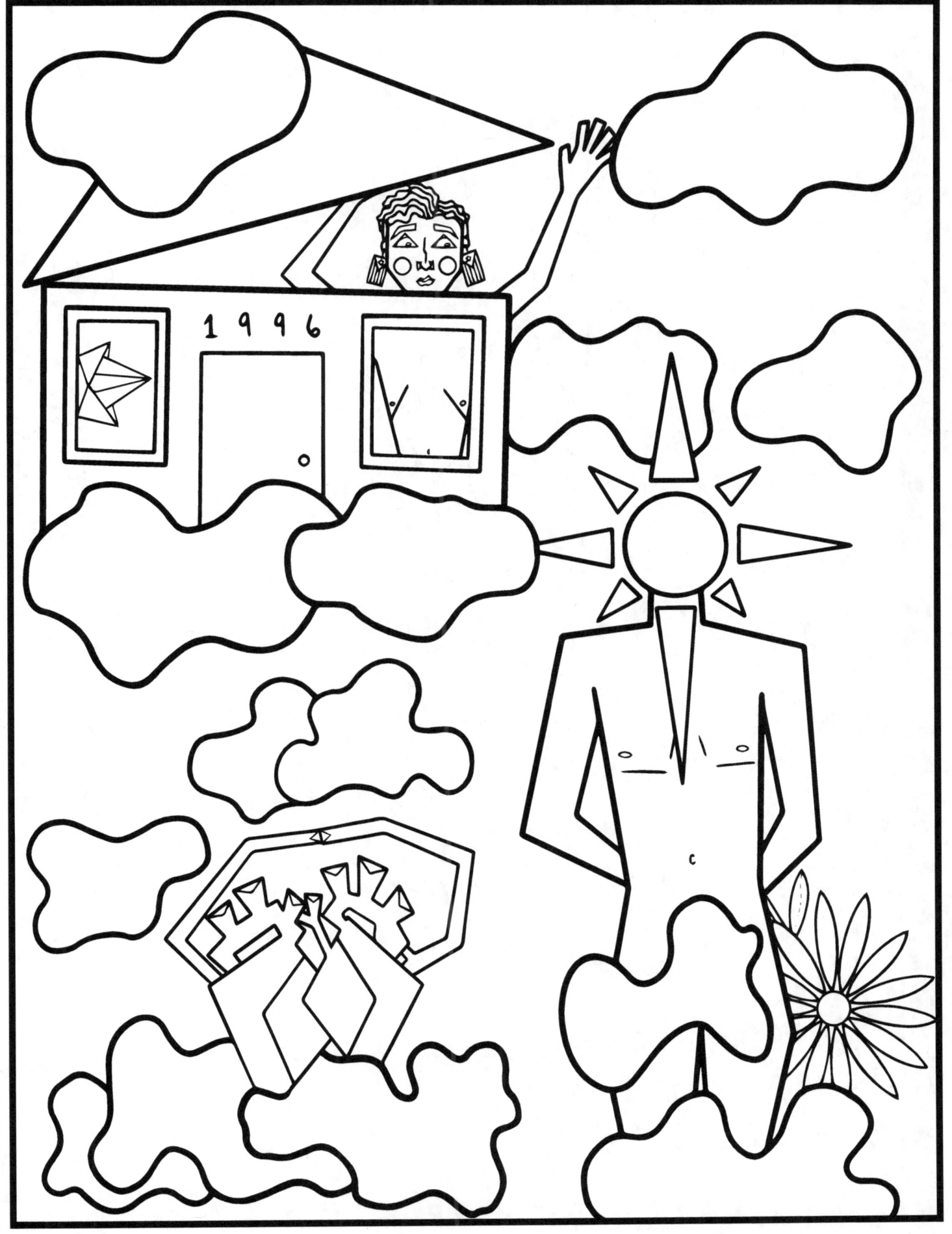

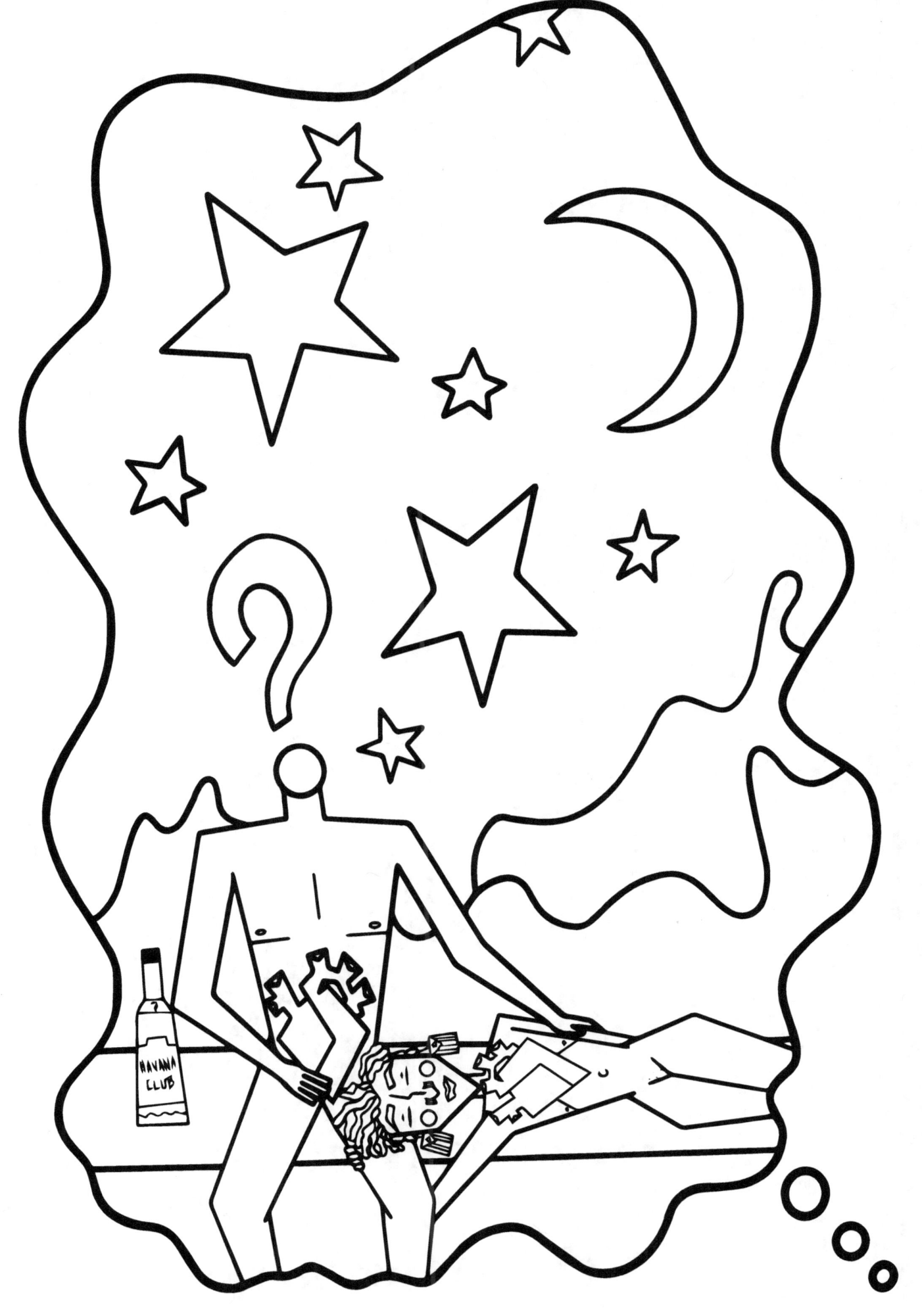

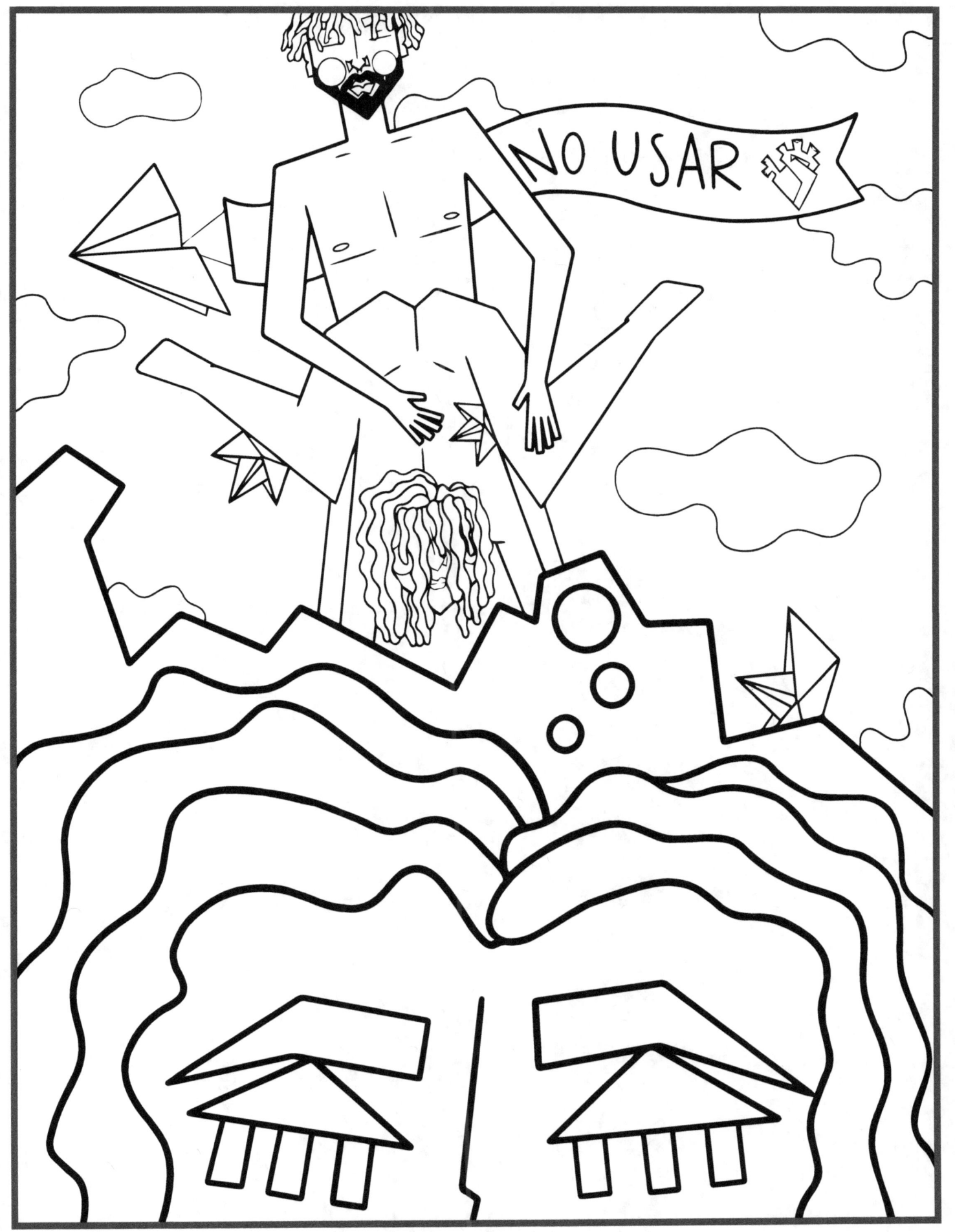

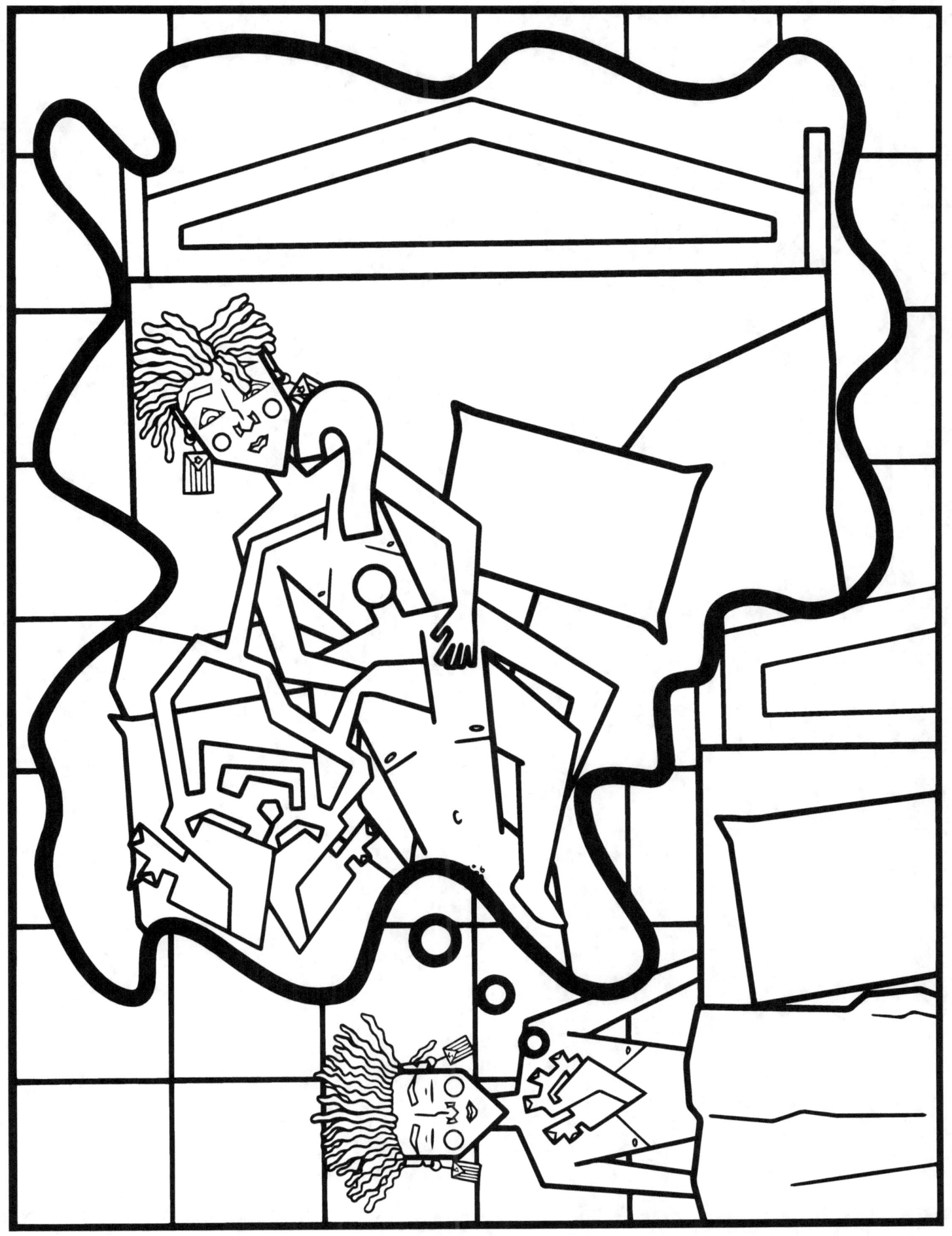

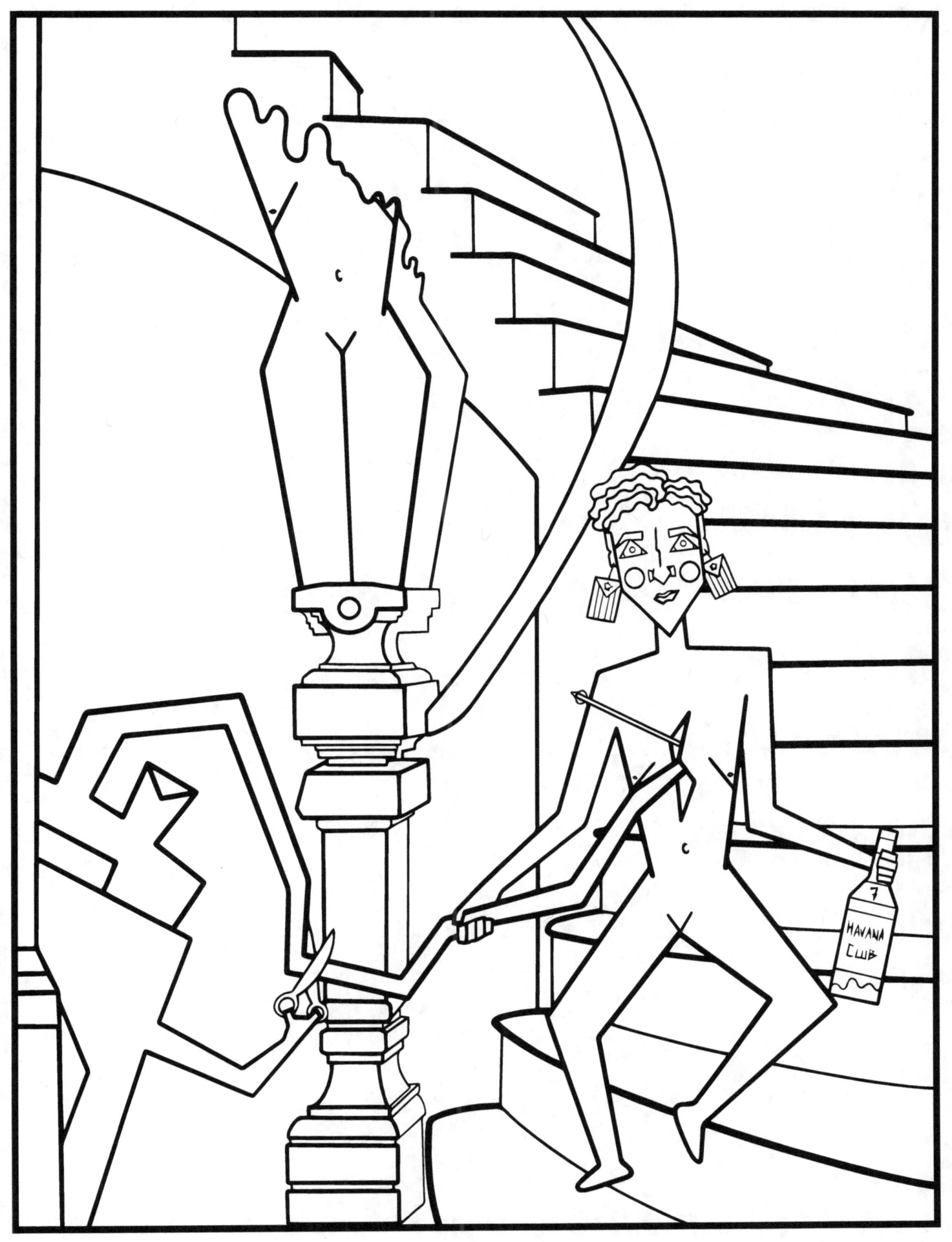

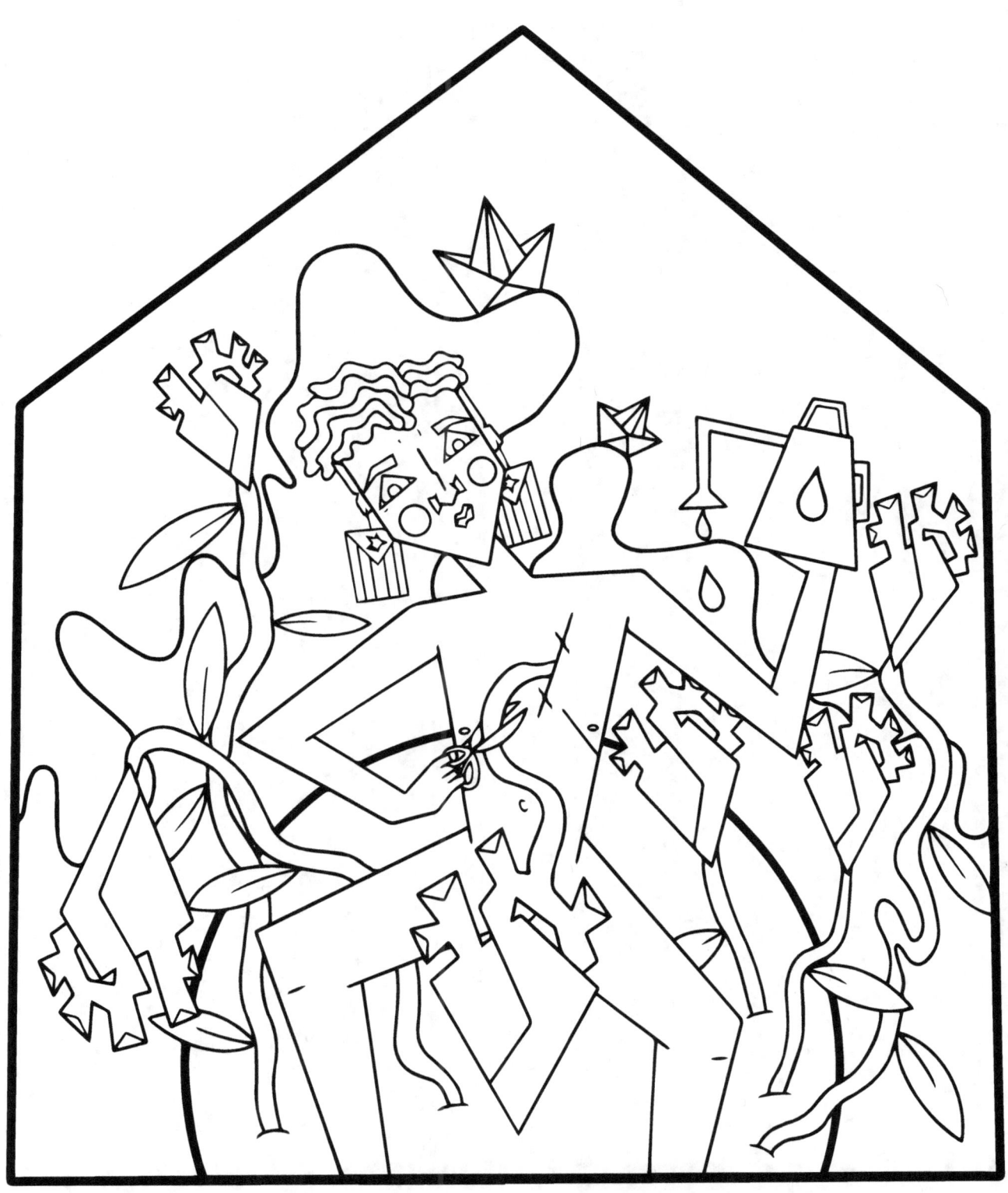

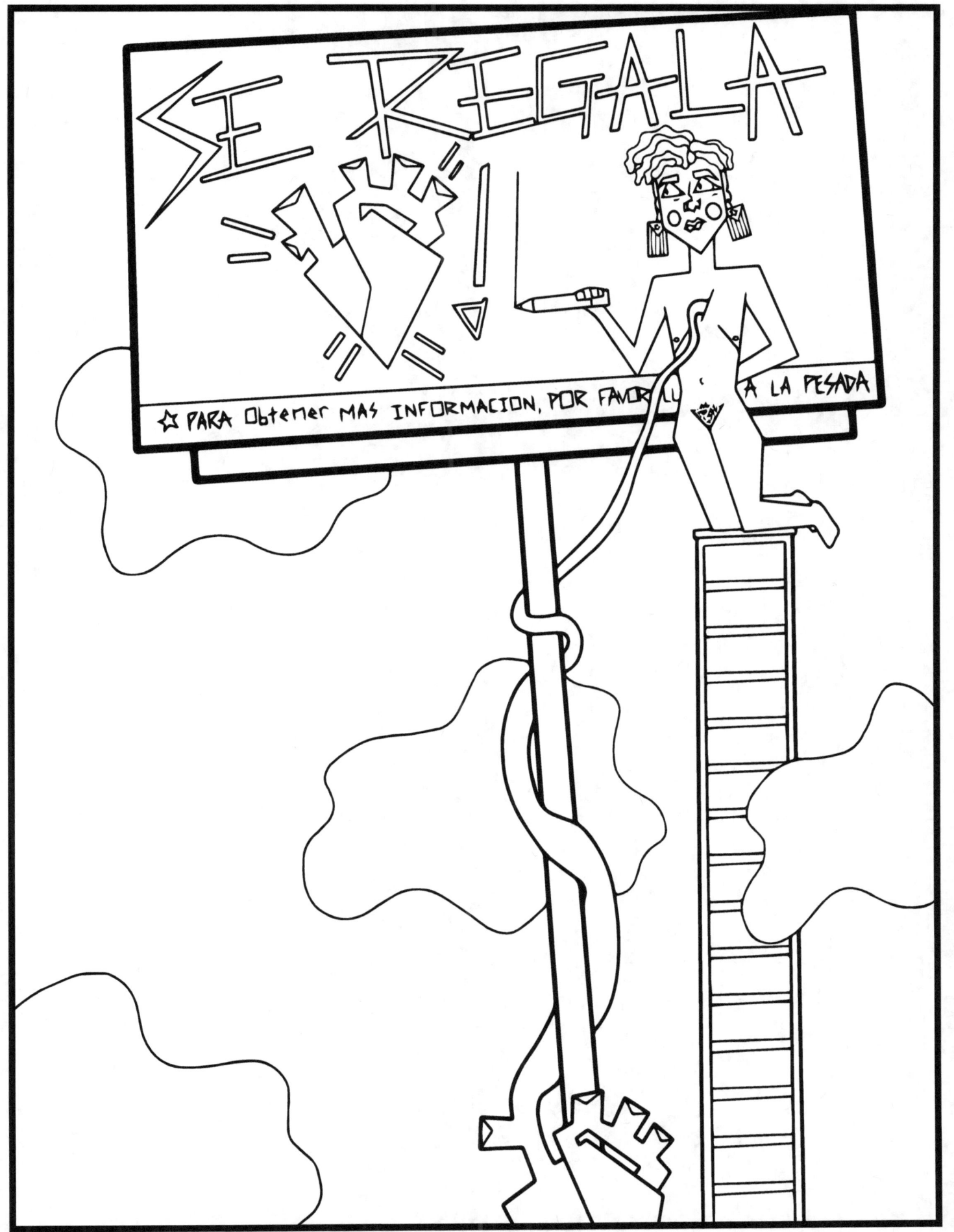

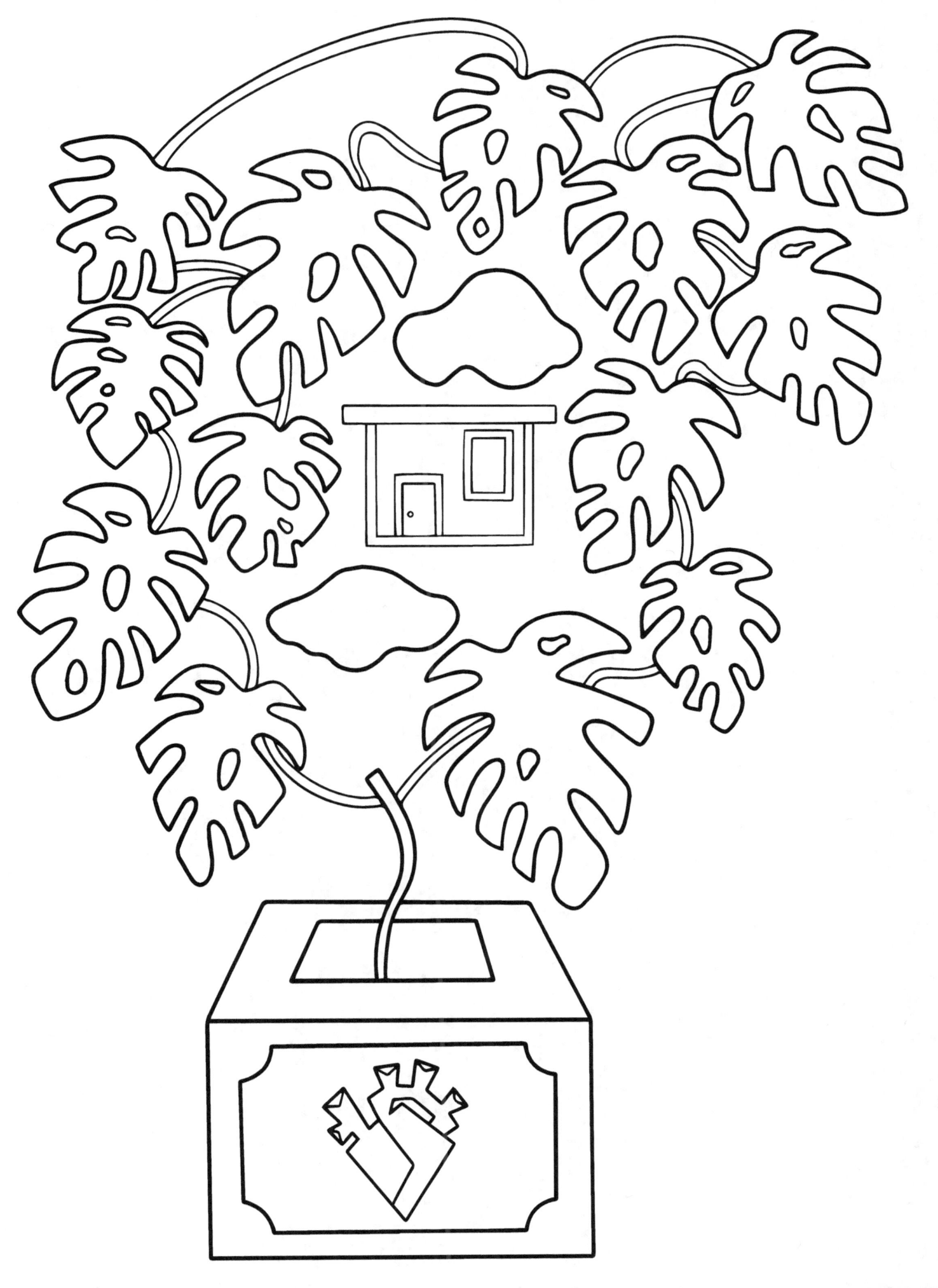

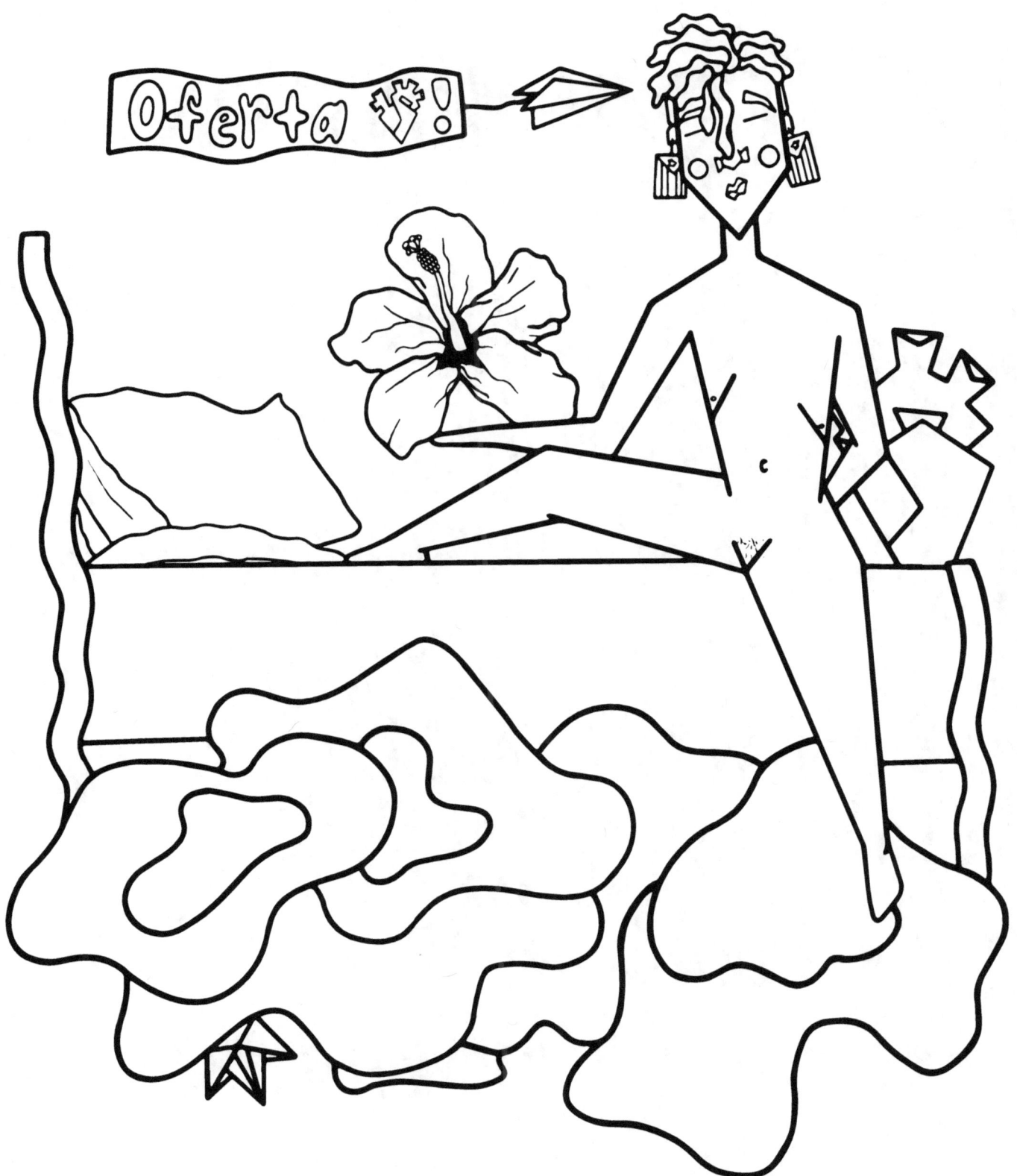

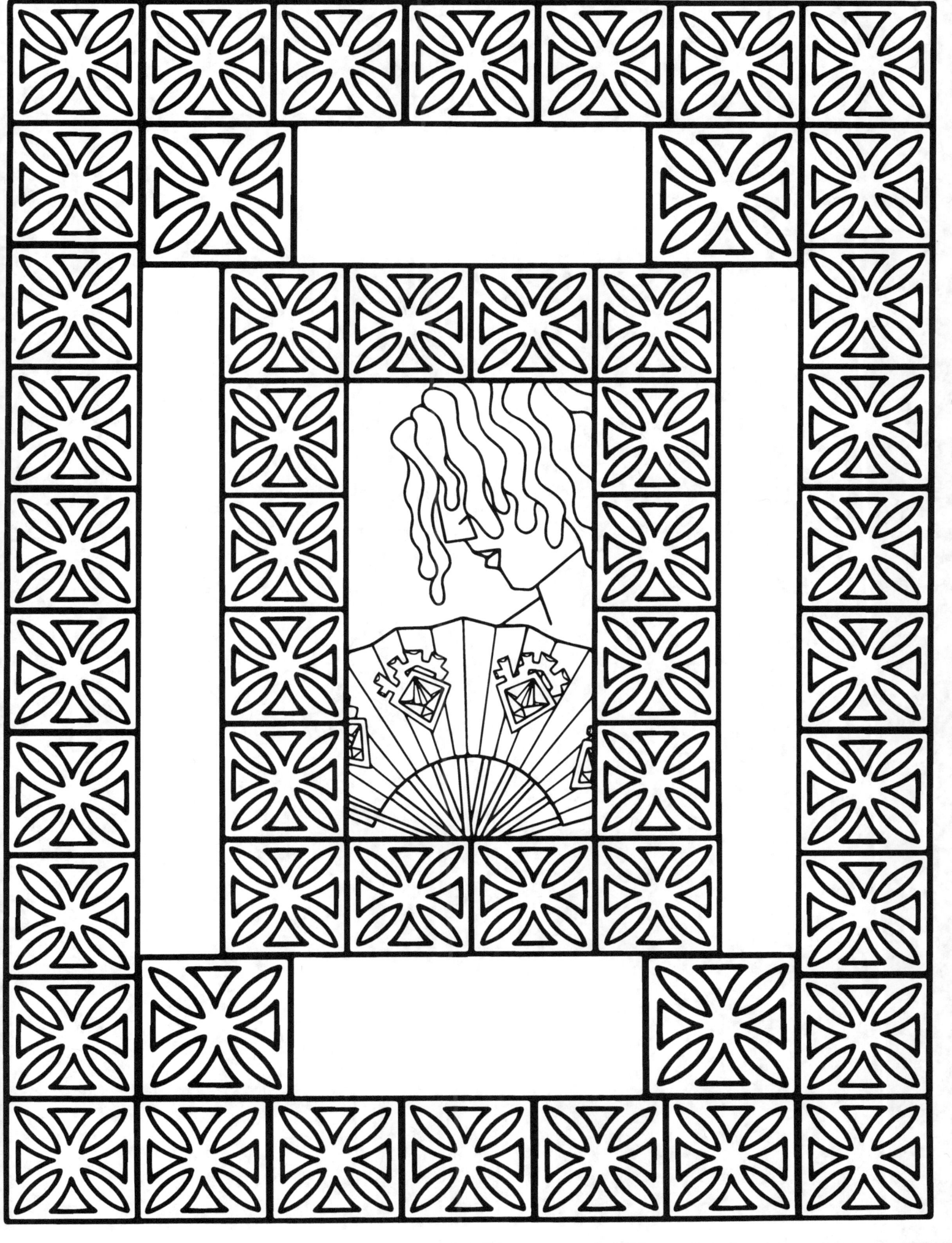

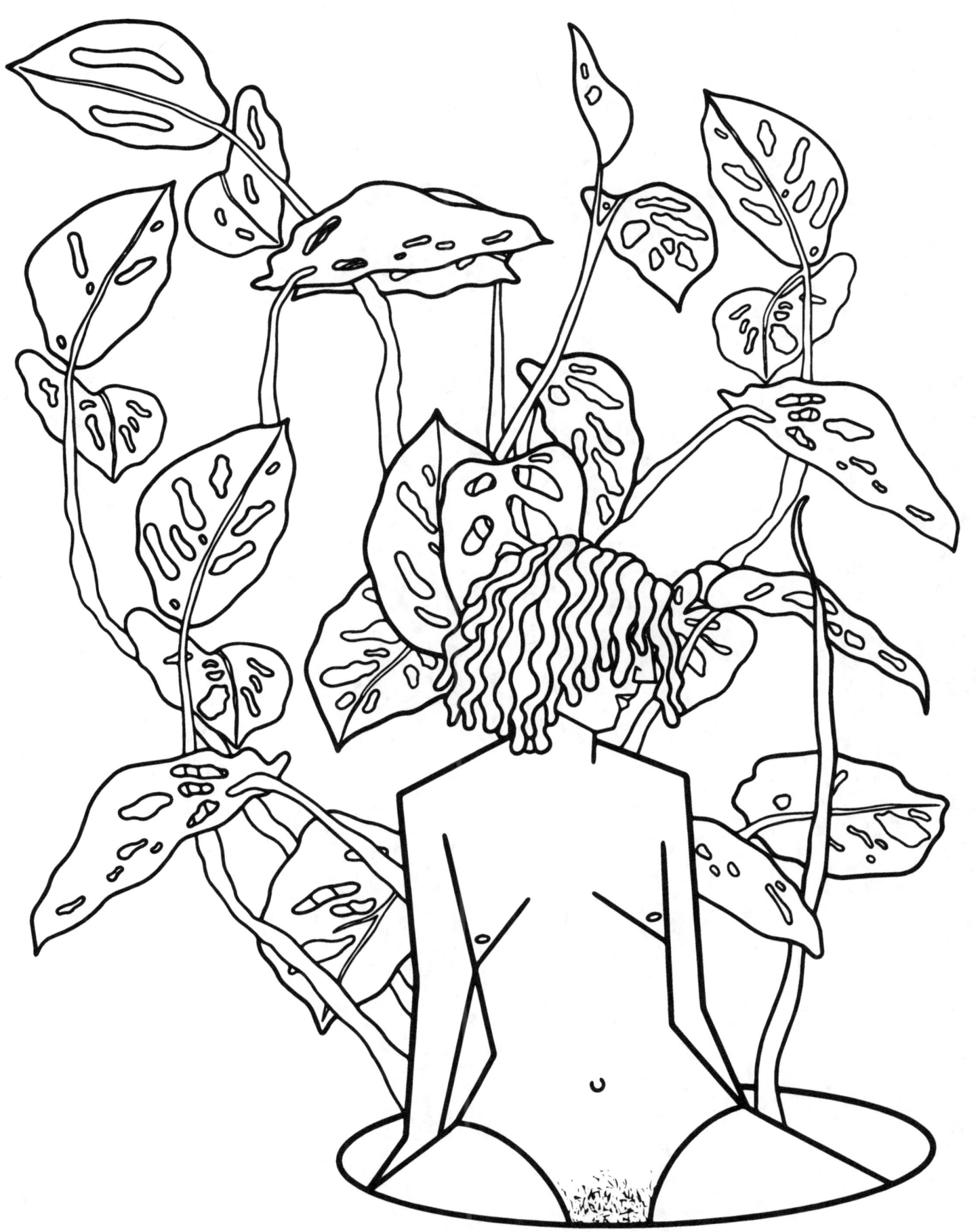

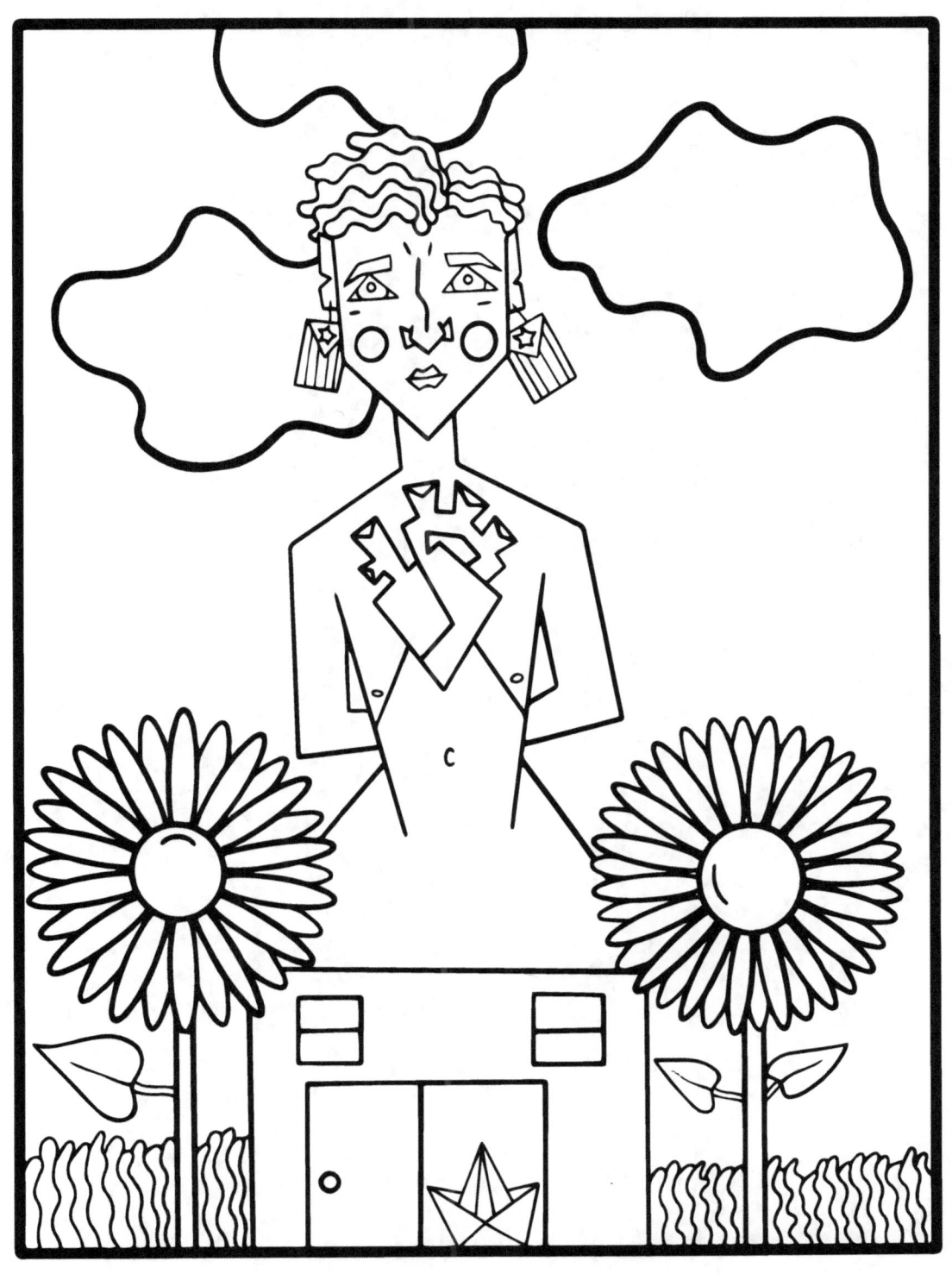